HASHIMOTO RECIPES COOKBOOK

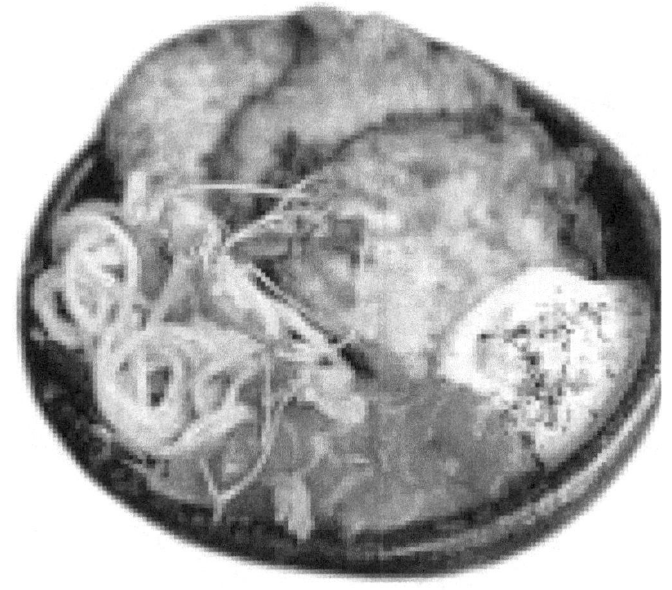

Simple Recipes and Meal Plan To Reverse

Thyroid Gland Condition for Healthy Living

Isabelle Hartley

Copyright © 2023 By [Isabelle Hartley]

All content in this book is protected under copyright laws. Any reproduction, distribution, or unauthorized use of any part of this book without the prior written consent of the copyright owner is strictly prohibited except for personal use.

OTHER BOOKS BY THIS AUTHOR

1. RECIPES FOR LOW BLOOD CHOLESTEROL
2. ATKINS DIET RECIPES COOKBOOK
3. CARDIAC DISEASE DIET COOKBOOK
4. CELIAC DISEASE RECIPES COOKBOOK
5. JUICING RECIPES FOR CANCER
6. LOW SUGAR DIET GUIDE FOR BEGINNERS

TABLE OF CONTENTS

Introduction vii

Chapter 1 ix

Types of Hashimoto's Disease: ix

Causes of Hashimoto's Disease:.....................................ix

Symptoms of Hashimoto's Disease: x

Diagnosis and Treatment: xii

Managing Hashimoto's Disease:....................................xii

Chapter 2 xiv

Foods to Include:..xiv

Foods to Avoid:...xv

Benefits xvii

How to follow Hashimoto diet.......................................xxi

Complications xxiv

CHAPTER 3: BREAKFAST RERCIPES xxviii

1. Quinoa Breakfast Bowl: xxviii

2. Sweet Potato Hash with Eggs:...............................xxviii

3. Greek Yogurt Parfait:...xxix

4. Avocado and Smoked Salmon Toast: xxx

5. Spinach and Mushroom Omelette:.................................xxx

6. Banana Nut Overnight Oats:......................................xxxi

7. Coconut Berry Smoothie Bowl:...................................xxxi

8. Turmeric Ginger Smoothie: xxxii

9. Chia Seed Pudding:..xxxiii

10. Cauliflower and Kale Breakfast Bowl:.......................xxxiii

CHAPTER 4: LUNCH RECIPES xxxv

1. Quinoa and Roasted Vegetable Salad: xxxv

2. Salmon and Avocado Wrap: xxxv

3. Vegetarian Lentil Soup: xxxvi

Chicken and Quinoa Bowl:...xxxvii

5. Mushroom and Spinach Omelette: xxxvii

6. Turkey and Avocado Lettuce Wraps: xxxviii

7. Quinoa Stuffed Bell Peppers:....................................xxxix

8. Chickpea and Spinach Curry: xxxix

9. Eggplant and Tomato Quinoa Bowl: xl

10. Shrimp and Vegetable Stir-Fry:................................xli

CHAPTER 5: DINNER RECIPES xlii

1. Baked Salmon with Lemon-Dill Sauce: xlii

2. Cauliflower and Chickpea Curry:.....................................xliii

3. Turkey and Vegetable Stir-Fry:.....................................xliii

4. Quinoa and Black Bean Stuffed Peppers:.......................xliv

5. Chicken and Vegetable Skewers:..................................xlv

6. Sweet Potato and Kale Hash:.......................................xlv

7. Vegetarian Quinoa Paella: xlvi

8. Baked Chicken with Garlic and Rosemary:...................xlvii

9. Sesame Ginger Salmon Bowl: xlvii

10. Mushroom and Spinach Stuffed Chicken Breast:.........xlviii

CHAPTER 6: SNACK AND DESSERT RECIPES l

1. Energy-Boosting Nut Mix: l

2. Greek Yogurt and Berry Parfait:...................................l

3. Avocado Chocolate Mousse: li

4. Baked Apple Slices with Cinnamon:..............................lii

5. Coconut Chia Seed Pudding: lii

Conclusion...liv

CONTACT US 1

FREE 30DAYS MEAL PLANNER.......................................3

Introduction

I wanted to start this book with honoring James, a common man with an amazing tale of perseverance, fortitude, and how a well-balanced diet can transform lives. James had always been concerned about his health, but as the years went by, he started to exhibit a number of odd symptoms. His complexion looked to have lost its healthy glow, his hair was thinning, and fatigue dragged him down like a thick blanket. James underwent numerous examinations and trips to the doctor before learning he had Hashimoto's illness, which drastically altered his life.

Determined to regain control of his health, James delved into extensive research about Hashimoto's disease and discovered the profound impact of diet on autoimmune conditions. He decided to take matters into his own hands and committed to a journey of culinary exploration, crafting meals that not only satisfied his taste buds but also nourished his body in its fight against the autoimmune disorder.

Equipped with a fresh understanding of nutrition, James adopted the Hashimoto diet, emphasizing meals high in nutrients and avoiding those that would worsen his illness. He turned his kitchen into a laboratory, experimenting with different components to find the ideal ratio to bolster his immune system.

James noted small changes throughout the course of the weeks. His energy returned, and the lingering shroud of exhaustion started to clear. His cheeks took on color again, and his hair began to grow back in thickness.

James's journey transformed his own life through the simple act of choosing the right ingredients and savoring every bite, James proved that sometimes, the most powerful medicine can be found on our plates.

Chapter 1

An autoimmune condition affecting the thyroid gland is Hashimoto's disease, sometimes referred to as Hashimoto's thyroiditis. This illness, named for the Japanese physician Hakaru Hashimoto, was originally reported in 1912 and is characterized by an immune system attack on the thyroid that results in inflammation and eventually damages thyroid tissue. The thyroid gland is a key player in metabolism regulation because it produces hormones that affect many different body processes.

Types of Hashimoto's Disease:

There is one primary type of Hashimoto's disease:

1. Hashimoto's Hypothyroidism: The most prevalent kind of Hashimoto's illness causes an underactive thyroid. Hypothyroidism results from the thyroid gland's decreased ability to produce thyroid hormones as a result of immune system injury to the thyroid tissue.

Causes of Hashimoto's Disease:

Although the precise causation of Hashimoto's illness is unknown, it is thought to be the result of a confluence of environmental and hereditary variables. Among the crucial elements are:

1. Genetics: Hashimoto's illness is more common in people with a family history of autoimmune diseases, especially thyroid conditions. People may be predisposed to autoimmune diseases by specific genes.

2. Gender: Hashimoto's disease is more common in women than in men. The reasons for this gender disparity are not completely clear, but hormonal factors may play a role.

3. Age: Though it can strike anyone at any age, Hashimoto's disease is typically discovered in people between the ages of 40 and 60. But it can also have an impact on kids and teenagers.

4. Other Autoimmune Conditions: Individuals who already suffer from other autoimmune disorders, such type 1 diabetes or rheumatoid arthritis, may be more susceptible to Hashimoto's disease.

5. Environmental Triggers: Some environmental variables can cause or worsen Hashimoto's disease in susceptible people. Examples include radiation exposure, excessive iodine exposure, and viral infections.

Symptoms of Hashimoto's Disease:

Hashimoto's disease symptoms can differ greatly from person to person and may appear gradually over time. Typical symptoms consist of:

1. Fatigue: One of the most common signs of Hashimoto's illness is chronic fatigue. People frequently experience fatigue, sluggishness, and difficulties sustaining their energy levels.

2. Weight Gain: Unexplained weight gain, even with reduced calorie intake, is a common symptom of an underactive thyroid.

3. Sensitivity to Cold: Individuals who have Hashimoto's disease may have particularly cold hands and feet and a heightened sensitivity to cold temperatures.

4. Dry Skin and Hair: The hair may become brittle and thin, and the skin may get pale and dry. Furthermore, hair loss could happen.

5. Muscle Weakness and Joint Pain: Hashimoto's disease can lead to muscle weakness and joint pain, making simple activities more challenging.

6. Constipation: Constipation and slow bowel movements are frequent signs of an underactive thyroid.

7. Depression and Mood Changes: Changes in mood, including depression and anxiety, are often associated with Hashimoto's disease.

8. Menstrual Irregularities: Menstrual periods in women with Hashimoto's disease may be erratic.

9. Swelling of the Thyroid (Goiter): In some cases, the thyroid gland may become enlarged, leading to a visible swelling in the neck.

10. Elevated Cholesterol Levels: Increased cholesterol can be a symptom of hypothyroidism and raise the risk of cardiac problems.

Diagnosis and Treatment:

A patient's medical history, physical examination, thyroid function tests, and antibodies linked to the illness are usually used in the diagnosis of Hashimoto's disease. Thyroid hormone replacement medication, often in the form of synthetic thyroid hormones like levothyroxine, is the primary treatment for Hashimoto's disease. This drug aids in symptom relief and thyroid hormone normalization.

Managing Hashimoto's Disease:

Although medication is an essential part of treating Hashimoto's disease, lifestyle choices can have a big impact on general health. The following are some lifestyle factors to take into account for those with Hashimoto's disease:

1. Nutrition: For the thyroid to function properly, a diet that is well-balanced and contains enough iodine and selenium is essential. Dietary changes that eliminate gluten or dairy products

have been shown to help manage symptoms in certain people, so these lifestyle changes may be beneficial for them.

2. Stress Management: Chronic stress can exacerbate autoimmune conditions. Implementing stress-reduction techniques such as meditation, yoga, and deep breathing exercises can be beneficial.

3. Regular Exercise: Frequent physical activity can enhance mood, increase energy levels, and promote general wellbeing.

4. Adequate Sleep: Prioritizing sufficient and quality sleep is crucial for individuals with Hashimoto's disease, as it contributes to overall health and helps manage fatigue.

5. Regular Monitoring: Effective management requires routine follow-up visits with medical professionals, who can also monitor thyroid hormone levels and make necessary drug adjustments.

To sum up, Hashimoto's disease is an intricate autoimmune disorder that necessitates all-encompassing care. An essential first step in managing Hashimoto's illness is to comprehend its forms, causes, and symptoms. People with Hashimoto's disease can live happy, productive lives and appropriately manage their health with the correct medical care, lifestyle changes, and supportive community.

Chapter 2

The goals of a Hashimoto diet are to manage the symptoms of Hashimoto's disease, an autoimmune disorder that affects the thyroid gland, and to promote thyroid health. There are general guidelines for things to include and avoid in a Hashimoto diet in order to attain optimal health, even though individual dietary demands may vary

Foods to Include:

1. Nutrient-Dense Whole Foods: Prioritize in your diet the consumption of entire, nutrient-dense foods such as fruits, vegetables, lean meats, and whole grains. These foods' essential vitamins, minerals, and antioxidants support overall wellness.

2. Lean Proteins: Include lean protein sources such tofu, beans, lentils, fish, and fowl. Maintaining a healthy metabolism and enhancing muscular health require protein.

3. Healthy Fats: Add healthy fat-containing foods such as avocados, nuts, seeds, and olive oil. These lipids are necessary for both the manufacturing of hormones and overall cellular activity.

4. Iodine-Rich Foods: Verify that you're getting the right amount of iodine—not too much. While iodine is essential for thyroid function, excessive iodine intake may be problematic for

people with Hashimoto's disease. Consume iodine-rich foods in moderation, such as dairy, seafood, and seaweed.

5. Selenium-Rich Foods: Selenium is a trace mineral that plays a role in thyroid function and can have anti-inflammatory effects. Good sources of selenium include Brazil nuts, seafood, and lean meats.

6. Fiber-Rich Foods: Include plenty of fiber from fruits, vegetables, and whole grains to support digestive health and maintain stable blood sugar levels.

7. Gluten-Free Options: Some individuals with Hashimoto's disease may benefit from a gluten-free diet. Gluten can be inflammatory for some people, and eliminating it may alleviate symptoms. Choose gluten-free grains like quinoa, rice, and gluten-free oats.

8. Probiotic-Rich Foods: Support gut health with probiotic-rich foods such as yogurt, kefir, sauerkraut, and kimchi. A healthy gut microbiome is linked to overall wellbeing and may positively impact autoimmune conditions.

Foods to Avoid:

1. Excessive Iodine: Iodine is required for thyroid function, but too much of it can cause or worsen Hashimoto's illness. Restrict

your consumption of iodized salt and foods high in iodine, such seaweed.

2. Processed Foods and Sugars: Reduce the amount of processed meals and added sugars you eat. These may have a detrimental effect on general health and exacerbate inflammation.

3. Gluten: Since some people with Hashimoto's disease may be gluten sensitive, you may want to think about cutting back on or removing gluten from your diet. Gluten may exacerbate inflammation in those who are sensitive to it.

4. Soy Products: There are substances in soy that could affect thyroid function. Although moderate soy consumption might not be detrimental for everyone, those with Hashimoto's disease should be cautious about how much soy they eat.

5. Cruciferous Vegetables (in Excess): Despite being high in nutrients, some veggies also contain substances that, in excess, may disrupt thyroid function. It's usually advised to cook cruciferous veggies or to eat them in moderation.

6. Dairy (for Some): Dairy may cause sensitivities in certain Hashimoto's disease patients. If you can handle it, go for premium, fermented dairy products or investigate dairy-free options.

7. Alcohol and Caffeine: Limit your intake of alcohol and caffeine because these substances can cause sleep disturbances and stress, both of which can make symptoms worse.

8. Artificial Additives: Steer clear of foods that have artificial coloring, preservatives, or additives as these might aggravate inflammation and have a detrimental effect on general health.

To customize their diet to meet their unique needs, people with Hashimoto's disease are encouraged to work closely with medical specialists and think about speaking with a qualified dietitian. Maintaining a food journal and observing the impact of various foods on symptoms might yield important information about personal nutritional needs. With Hashimoto's disease, achieving optimal health requires a tailored approach to lifestyle, diet, and medication.

Starting a Hashimoto diet for beginners can have a number of fundamental advantages, including treating Hashimoto's disease and enhancing general health. The following are the main benefits for anyone beginning this journey:

Benefits

1. **Supports Thyroid Function:** Supporting the health of the thyroid gland is the main objective of a Hashimoto diet. People with Hashimoto's disease can contribute to maintaining healthy

thyroid function by consuming nutrient-dense foods and avoiding possible triggers. This is necessary to control energy levels, metabolism, and other body processes.

2. Reduces Inflammation: In order to lessen inflammation in the body, the Hashimoto diet includes a number of anti-inflammatory foods and steers clear of things that may irritate the body, such as gluten. Reducing chronic inflammation can help with symptom relief and enhance general health as it is frequently linked to autoimmune disorders.

3. Balances Blood Sugar Levels: The Hashimoto diet places a strong emphasis on fiber, complex carbs, and well-balanced meals, all of which can aid with blood sugar stabilization. This is especially crucial for those who have Hashimoto's disease because blood sugar swings can affect mood and energy levels.

4. Promotes Gut Health: Good digestion is associated with general health and may be involved in autoimmune diseases. A balanced and healthy gut flora can be achieved with the Hashimoto diet, which emphasizes gut-friendly options and foods high in probiotics.

5. Enhances Nutrient Intake: Consuming nutrient-dense whole foods that are high in vitamins, minerals, and antioxidants is encouraged by the diet. Sufficient nutritional consumption promotes general health and can assist in addressing any shortages that people with Hashimoto's disease may encounter.

6. **Manages Weight and Metabolism:** Those with Hashimoto's disease frequently struggle to reach and maintain a healthy weight, especially considering the possibility of weight gain associated with an underactive thyroid. The Hashimoto diet can help maintain a healthy metabolism and aid in weight management because of its emphasis on portion control and balanced nutrition.

7. **Enhances Energy Levels:** People who have Hashimoto's disease frequently feel exhausted and have low energy. By giving the body the nutrition it requires for long-lasting vitality, the Hashimoto diet seeks to alleviate these symptoms. Increased vitality can be attained through selecting foods that improve energy and balancing macronutrients.

8. **Encourages Mindful Eating:** A Hashimoto diet encourages mindful eating practices. A better connection with food is achieved through making thoughtful decisions, paying attention to signals of hunger and satiety, and being aware of the nutritional value of meals. Beyond the plate, this attention can have a favorable influence on general lifestyle decisions.

9. **Addresses Individual Sensitivities:** The Hashimoto diet acknowledges that people could react differently to different meals. People can alter their diets to suit their individual demands by observing how different foods affect their symptoms. Using a customized approach is essential to maximizing health results.

10. **Fosters a Positive Community:** Participating in the Hashimoto diet frequently entails reaching out to a group of people who are encouraging and going through similar struggles. On the path to improved health, exchanging stories, recipes, and advice creates a sense of community and offers priceless emotional support.

For those who are just learning about the Hashimoto diet, the main advantages go beyond just treating symptoms; they include a whole-person approach to wellness. People can empower themselves to manage the intricacies of Hashimoto's illness and work towards optimal wellbeing by embracing nutrient-rich foods, reducing potential triggers, and adopting mindful eating practices. Beginners should speak with medical specialists or qualified dietitians before making any dietary changes to ensure a safe and efficient approach to controlling Hashimoto's disease through nutrition.

A Hashimoto diet entails adopting deliberate and conscientious food choices to maintain thyroid function and control symptoms of Hashimoto's disease, an autoimmune disorder that affects the thyroid gland. Here is a how-to guide for implementing the Hashimoto diet:

How to follow Hashimoto diet

1. Educate Yourself: Spend some time learning about the Hashimoto's disease and its nutritional requirements before beginning the diet. Recognize the function of the thyroid gland, the ways in which autoimmune reactions influence it, and the possible links between Hashimoto's disease and specific foods.

2. Consult with Healthcare Professionals: Before making major dietary changes, it is imperative to contact with healthcare professionals such as registered dietitians and endocrinologists. These experts can offer tailored guidance based on your unique health demands and assist in creating a diet that meets your specific needs.

3. Identify Trigger Foods: Identify food triggers that can make symptoms worse. Dairy, soy, and gluten are common causes. To monitor the effects of various foods on your mood, energy level, and general well-being, keep a food journal.

4. Prioritize Nutrient-Dense Foods: Make sure you are getting enough vitamins and minerals by concentrating on complete meals that are high in nutrients. Incorporate lean meats, whole grains, healthy fats, and a range of vibrant fruits and vegetables into your meals. These foods boost thyroid function and offer the fundamentals for general wellness.

5. Consider Gluten-Free Options: Several Hashimoto's disease sufferers find relief by switching to a gluten-free diet. Wheat, barley, and rye all contain gluten, which some individuals find inflammatory. Look into rice, quinoa, and gluten-free oats as gluten-free substitutes.

6. Include Lean Proteins: Add sources of lean protein such fish, poultry, beans, lentils, and tofu. A balanced metabolism and the health of muscles depend on protein.

7. Manage Iodine Intake: Iodine is essential for thyroid function, but too much of it might cause issues for those who have Hashimoto's illness. Steer clear of excessive iodine supplementation and opt for foods high in iodine, such as dairy, fish, and seaweed, in moderation.

8. Balance Macronutrients: Every meal should have a macronutrient distribution that is well-balanced, with proteins, carbs, and fats. Maintaining a balance between these elements

promotes general energy levels and aids in blood sugar stabilization.

9. Restrict Sugar and Processed Food Intake: Reduce the amount of processed meals and added sugars you consume. These may have a detrimental effect on thyroid function and lead to inflammation. Pick complete, unprocessed foods whenever you can.

10. Watch Cruciferous Vegetables: Although cruciferous vegetables are high in nutrients, such as broccoli, cauliflower, and Brussels sprouts, eating too much of these can affect thyroid function. To lessen their goitrogenic qualities, cook these veggies.

11. Include Healthy Fats: Include foods like avocados, almonds, seeds, and olive oil that are good sources of fat. The synthesis of hormones and general cellular function depend on these lipids.

12. Stay Hydrated: Maintain proper hydration and general health throughout the day by consuming a sufficient amount of water. In addition to being beneficial for metabolic processes, enough hydration can help control symptoms like weariness.

13. Monitor Symptoms: Observe how various foods impact your symptoms. If you observe patterns of discomfort or

symptom aggravation following the consumption of particular foods, you may want to remove or minimize them from your diet.

14. Practice Mindful Eating: Embrace mindful eating by paying attention to your body's signals of hunger and fullness, being present throughout meals, and enjoying every bite. A healthy relationship with food is fostered and general welfare is enhanced via mindful eating.

15. Engage in Community Support: Make connections with people who are on the Hashimoto diet. Participate in online forums, communities, or support groups to learn from others on a similar path, exchange recipes, and share experiences.

To adhere to a Hashimoto diet, one must possess knowledge, self-awareness, and a dedication to making deliberate food decisions. People with Hashimoto's disease can optimize their diet to support thyroid function and improve overall wellbeing by working closely with healthcare providers, recognizing their unique triggers, and incorporating nutrient-dense foods. It's crucial to implement dietary changes gradually, pay attention to how your body reacts, and make any adjustments under the supervision of medical professionals.

Complications

Improper management of Hashimoto's disease can result in a number of consequences, some of which can be exacerbated by an improper diet. To lessen these difficulties, it is imperative that people with Hashimoto's disease follow a supportive diet. When the proper diet is not followed, the following possible issues could occur:

1. Hypothyroidism: Untreated or improperly managed Hashimoto's disease can lead to hypothyroidism, or an underactive thyroid. This happens as a result of the thyroid gland being attacked and damaged by the immune system, which lowers the thyroid hormone production. Numerous symptoms, such as lethargy, weight gain, cold sensitivity, and cognitive decline, can be brought on by hypothyroidism.

2. Goiter: An growth of the thyroid gland, known as a goiter, can arise from the chronic inflammation and damage resulting from Hashimoto's disease. The thyroid gland may grow noticeably enlarged if it is not properly managed with medication and dietary changes. This can cause discomfort and perhaps cause issues with breathing or swallowing.

3. Cardiovascular Issues: Heart problems may arise from hypothyroidism brought on by Hashimoto's illness. Untreated hypothyroidism is frequently associated with elevated levels of

LDL cholesterol and triglycerides, which raise the risk of atherosclerosis and heart disease. To reduce these risks, it is imperative to adopt a heart-healthy diet.

4. Mental Health Challenges: Untreated Hashimoto's disease may be a factor in mental health issues like anxiety and sadness. An imbalance in thyroid hormones can affect mood, cognitive function, and general mental health since thyroid hormones are essential for brain function.

5. Infertility and Menstrual Irregularities: Untreated Hashimoto's disease in women can cause irregular menstruation and, in rare circumstances, infertility. Hypothyroidism-related hormonal abnormalities can impact the reproductive system and make it difficult for women to become pregnant.

6. Myxedema Coma (Severe Hypothyroidism): Untreated severe hypothyroidism can, however infrequently, result in myxedema coma, a potentially fatal illness. Extreme symptoms like cold, disorientation, and respiratory failure indicate a medical emergency. To avoid such serious consequences, proper management of Hashimoto's disease is essential and includes both medicine and a supportive diet.

7. Peripheral Neuropathy: Peripheral neuropathy, which could result from hypothyroidism linked to Hashimoto's illness, can

cause symptoms like tingling, numbness, and weakness in the extremities. To lessen these issues, a diet that is well-balanced and promotes nerve health is crucial.

8. Pregnancy Complications: Untreated or poorly managed Hashimoto's illness during pregnancy increases the chance of many difficulties, such as miscarriage, premature birth, and problems with the unborn child's development. An eating plan that supports a healthy thyroid is essential for controlling Hashimoto's during pregnancy.

9. Joint Pain and Muscular Discomfort: Muscle rigidity and joint discomfort can both be attributed to hypothyroidism. The general quality of life and mobility may be affected by these symptoms. Changing to an anti-inflammatory diet could make these aches go away.

10. Cognitive Impairment: The function of the thyroid gland is vital to cognitive processes. Idiopathic hypothyroidism caused by Hashimoto's disease can impair cognition and cause memory problems and concentration problems.

If untreated, Hashimoto's disease can have major consequences, which emphasizes how crucial it is to follow the correct diet in order to control it. An essential part of overall care is a customized diet to maintain thyroid health, lower inflammation, and address potential nutritional shortages. Patients with Hashimoto's disease should collaborate closely with medical specialists, such as nutritionists and endocrinologists, to create a customized treatment plan that takes medication, dietary adjustments, and lifestyle changes into account. People can improve their overall quality of life and reduce the risk of complications by managing the disease proactively.

CHAPTER 3: BREAKFAST RERCIPES

These ten breakfast recipes are Hashimoto's friendly and use nutrient-dense ingredients to help with thyroid function. It is important to modify these recipes according to personal preferences and any particular dietary restrictions, as individual nutritional demands may differ:

1. Quinoa Breakfast Bowl:

Ingredients:

- 1 cup cooked quinoa
- 1/2 cup almond milk
- 1 tablespoon chia seeds
- 1/2 cup fresh berries (e.g., blueberries, raspberries)
- 1 tablespoon chopped nuts (e.g., almonds, walnuts)

Preparation:

1. Combine almond milk and cooked quinoa.
2. Add the chia seeds and stir, then let aside for a few minutes..
3. Top with fresh berries and chopped nuts.

2. Sweet Potato Hash with Eggs:

Ingredients:

- 1 medium sweet potato, grated

- 1 tablespoon olive oil

- 1/2 onion, diced

- 2 eggs

- Salt and pepper to taste

Preparation:

1. In olive oil, sauté diced onion and shredded sweet potato until they are soft.
2. Crack eggs into the wells you've made in the hash.
3. Cook the eggs until they are cooked through. Add pepper and salt for seasoning.

3. Greek Yogurt Parfait:

Ingredients:

- 1 cup Greek yogurt (or dairy-free alternative)

- 1/4 cup granola (gluten-free if necessary)

- 1/2 cup mixed berries

- 1 tablespoon honey or maple syrup

Preparation:

1. In a glass or bowl, arrange Greek yogurt, granola, and mixed berries.
2. Drizzle with maple syrup or honey.

4. *Avocado and Smoked Salmon Toast:*

Ingredients:

- 2 slices gluten-free or wholegrain bread
- 1/2 avocado, sliced
- 2 ounces smoked salmon
- Lemon juice
- Fresh dill for garnish

Preparation:

Toast the slices of bread.

Add smoked salmon and avocado slices on top.

Drizzle with freshly squeezed lemon juice and add some dill for garnish.

5. *Spinach and Mushroom Omelette:*

Ingredients:

- 3 eggs
- 1/2 cup fresh spinach, chopped
- 1/4 cup mushrooms, sliced
- 1 tablespoon olive oil
- Salt and pepper to taste

Preparation:

1. 1. Cook mushrooms in olive oil until they become soft.
2. 2. Cook the chopped spinach until it wilts.
3. 3. Beat eggs, cover vegetables with them, and cook until set. Season with salt and pepper.

6. Banana Nut Overnight Oats:

Ingredients:

- 1/2 cup rolled oats
- 1/2 cup almond milk
- 1/2 banana, mashed
- 1 tablespoon chia seeds
- 1 tablespoon chopped nuts (e.g., pecans, almonds)

Preparation:

1. In a jar, combine oats, almond milk, mashed banana, and chia seeds.

2. Keep chilled all night.

3. Before serving, sprinkle chopped nuts over top.

7. Coconut Berry Smoothie Bowl:

Ingredients:

- 1 cup coconut milk

- 1/2 cup frozen berries (e.g., strawberries, blueberries)

- 1/2 banana

- 1 tablespoon shredded coconut

- 1 tablespoon hemp seeds

Preparation:

1. Puree the banana, frozen berries, and coconut milk until smooth.

2. Transfer to a bowl and garnish with hemp seeds and shredded coconut.

8. Turmeric Ginger Smoothie:

Ingredients:

- 1 cup almond milk

- 1/2 teaspoon ground turmeric

- 1/2 teaspoon grated ginger

- 1/2 banana

- 1 tablespoon almond butter

Preparation:

1. Until smooth, blend almond milk, ginger, turmeric, banana, and almond butter.

9. Chia Seed Pudding:

Ingredients:

- 2 tablespoons chia seeds
- 1/2 cup coconut milk
- 1/2 teaspoon vanilla extract
- 1/2 cup mixed berries
- 1 tablespoon sliced almonds

Preparation:

1. In a container, combine the chia seeds, coconut milk, and vanilla extract.

2. Keep chilled for many hours or overnight.

3. Before serving, garnish with sliced almonds and a mixture of berries.

10. Cauliflower and Kale Breakfast Bowl:

Ingredients:

- 1 cup cauliflower rice
- 1 cup kale, chopped
- 1 tablespoon coconut oil
- 2 eggs
- Salt and pepper to taste

Preparation:

1. In coconut oil, sauté greens and cauliflower rice till soft.

2. Crack eggs into the wells you've made in the mixture.

3. Cook the eggs until they are cooked through. Add pepper and salt for seasoning.

For those on a Hashimoto diet, these recipes offer a range of delectable and nutritious options. Adapt ingredients and quantities to suit dietary requirements and personal tastes. Seek individual counsel from healthcare professionals at all times.

CHAPTER 4: LUNCH RECIPES

These ten nutrient-dense lunch meals are Hashimoto's friendly and will help your thyroid function. Don't forget to adjust these recipes to your specific tastes and dietary requirements:

1. Quinoa and Roasted Vegetable Salad:

Ingredients:

- 1 cup cooked quinoa
- Assorted roasted vegetables (e.g., bell peppers, zucchini, cherry tomatoes)
- 2 cups fresh spinach or kale
- Feta cheese (optional)
- Olive oil and balsamic vinegar for dressing

Preparation:

Combine cooked quinoa with fresh greens and roasted veggies.

Drizzle with balsamic vinegar and olive oil.

If preferred, sprinkle crumbled feta cheese on top.

2. Salmon and Avocado Wrap:

Ingredients:

- 1 grilled or baked salmon fillet

- 1 wholegrain or gluten-free wrap
- 1/2 avocado, sliced
- Mixed greens
- Lemon juice

Preparation:

1. Top the wrap with salmon, avocado, and mixed greens.

2. Drizzle with newly squeezed lemon juice.

3. Roll up and use a toothpick to fasten.

3. Vegetarian Lentil Soup:

Ingredients:

- 1 cup dry lentils, rinsed
- 1 onion, diced
- 2 carrots, chopped
- 2 celery stalks, chopped
- 4 cups vegetable broth
- 1 teaspoon cumin
- Salt and pepper to taste

Preparation:

1. Saute the onion, carrots, and celery in a pot until they are tender.

2. Include the cumin, lentils, and vegetable broth. Cook the lentils by simmering them.

3. Add pepper and salt for seasoning.

Chicken and Quinoa Bowl:

Ingredients:

- Grilled chicken breast, sliced
- 1 cup cooked quinoa
- Roasted broccoli and cauliflower
- 1/4 cup hummus
- Lemon-tahini dressing

Preparation:

1. Fill a bowl with quinoa, roasted veggies, and sliced chicken.

2. Include some hummus.

3. Add a lemon-tahini dressing drizzle.

5. Mushroom and Spinach Omelette:

Ingredients:

- 3 eggs
- 1/2 cup sliced mushrooms
- 1 cup fresh spinach

- 1 tablespoon olive oil
- Salt and pepper to taste

Preparation:

1. In olive oil, sauté the spinach and mushrooms until they wilt.

2. Whisk the eggs and add them to the vegetables. Cook until the mixture solidifies.

3. Add pepper and salt for seasoning.

6. *Turkey and Avocado Lettuce Wraps:*

Ingredients:

- Sliced turkey breast
- Large lettuce leaves (e.g., butter lettuce or romaine)
- 1/2 avocado, sliced
- Tomato slices
- Mustard or hummus for spreading

Preparation:

1. Arrange the lettuce leaves and arrange the turkey, avocado, and tomato in layers.
2. For extra taste, spread hummus or mustard.

3. Roll up and use toothpicks to fasten.

7. Quinoa Stuffed Bell Peppers:

Ingredients:

- Bell peppers, halved and cleaned
- 1 cup cooked quinoa
- Black beans, drained and rinsed
- Diced tomatoes
- Shredded cheese (optional)

Preparation:

1. Combine chopped tomatoes, black beans, and cooked quinoa.

2. Insert the mixture into bell pepper halves.

3. If preferred, sprinkle with cheese. Bake peppers until they become soft.

8. Chickpea and Spinach Curry:

Ingredients:

- 1 can chickpeas, drained
- 1 onion, finely chopped
- 2 tomatoes, diced

- 2 cups fresh spinach

- Coconut milk

- Curry spices (turmeric, cumin, coriander)

Preparation:

Add curry spices to a sautéed onion after it turns golden.

Add the tomatoes, coconut milk, and chickpeas. Simmer for the flavors to blend.

Cook the fresh spinach until it wilts.

9. Eggplant and Tomato Quinoa Bowl:

Ingredients:

- 1 cup cooked quinoa

- Roasted eggplant slices

- Cherry tomatoes, halved

- Kalamata olives, sliced

- Feta cheese (optional)

Preparation:

1. Mix together the quinoa, olives, cherry tomatoes, and roasted eggplant.

2. If desired, sprinkle crumbled feta over top.

10. Shrimp and Vegetable Stir-Fry:

Ingredients:

- Shrimp, peeled and deveined
- Broccoli florets
- Bell peppers, sliced
- Snow peas
- Tamari or gluten-free soy sauce

Preparation:

1. In a pan, stir-fry the bell peppers, broccoli, snow peas, and shrimp.

2. To add flavor, add soy sauce or tamari.

3. You can serve it with cauliflower rice or brown rice.

These lunch recipes offer a range of tasty and nutrient-dense options suitable for anyone on the Hashimoto diet. For individualized guidance, speak with medical professionals and modify the components and portions according to personal tastes and dietary requirements.

CHAPTER 5: DINNER RECIPES

Here are 10 Hashimoto-friendly dinner recipes designed to support thyroid health with nutrient-dense ingredients. As always, adjust these recipes based on personal preferences and dietary restrictions:

1. Baked Salmon with Lemon-Dill Sauce:

- Ingredients:

- Salmon fillets

- Lemon juice

- Fresh dill, chopped

- Olive oil

- Salt and pepper to taste

- Preparation:

1. Place salmon on a baking sheet.

2. Drizzle with olive oil and lemon juice, sprinkle with chopped dill, salt, and pepper.

3. Bake until salmon is cooked through.

2. Cauliflower and Chickpea Curry:

- Ingredients:

- Cauliflower florets
- Chickpeas, drained
- Onion, diced
- Tomato sauce
- Coconut milk
- Curry spices (cumin, coriander, turmeric)

- Preparation:

1. Sauté onion until soft, add curry spices.

2. Stir in cauliflower, chickpeas, tomato sauce, and coconut milk.

3. Simmer until cauliflower is tender.

3. Turkey and Vegetable Stir-Fry:

- Ingredients:

- Ground turkey

- Mixed vegetables (broccoli, bell peppers, carrots)

- Tamari or gluten-free soy sauce

- Garlic, minced

- Ginger, grated

- Preparation:

1. Cook ground turkey in a pan until browned.

2. Add mixed vegetables, garlic, and ginger. Stir-fry until vegetables are tender.

3. Season with tamari or soy sauce.

4. *Quinoa and Black Bean Stuffed Peppers:*

- Ingredients:

- Bell peppers, halved and cleaned

- Cooked quinoa

- Black beans, drained and rinsed

- Salsa

- Shredded cheese (optional)

- Preparation:

1. Mix quinoa, black beans, and salsa.

2. Stuff the mixture into halved bell peppers.

3. Sprinkle with cheese if desired. Bake until peppers are tender.

5. Chicken and Vegetable Skewers:

- Ingredients:

- Chicken breast, cut into chunks

- Cherry tomatoes

- Zucchini, sliced

- Red onion, cut into wedges

- Olive oil

- Lemon juice

- Preparation:

1. Thread chicken and vegetables onto skewers.

2. Drizzle with olive oil and lemon juice.

3. Grill or bake until chicken is cooked through.

6. Sweet Potato and Kale Hash:

- Ingredients:

- Sweet potatoes, diced

- Kale, chopped

- Red onion, diced

- Olive oil

- Paprika and cumin

- Preparation:

1. Sauté sweet potatoes and red onion in olive oil until tender.

2. Add chopped kale and spices. Cook until kale is wilted.

7. *Vegetarian Quinoa Paella:*

- Ingredients:

- Quinoa

- Vegetable broth

- Bell peppers, diced

- Cherry tomatoes, halved

- Artichoke hearts, quartered

- Saffron and paprika

- Preparation:

1. Cook quinoa in vegetable broth with saffron and paprika.

2. Stir in diced bell peppers, cherry tomatoes, and artichoke hearts.

8. Baked Chicken with Garlic and Rosemary:

- Ingredients:

- Chicken thighs or breasts

- Garlic, minced

- Fresh rosemary, chopped

- Olive oil

- Lemon zest

- Preparation:

1. Rub chicken with minced garlic, rosemary, olive oil, and lemon zest.

2. Bake until chicken is golden and cooked through.

9. Sesame Ginger Salmon Bowl:

- Ingredients:

- Salmon fillets

- Brown rice or cauliflower rice

- Steamed broccoli

- Sesame oil and soy sauce

- Fresh ginger, grated

- Preparation:

1. Grill or bake salmon with sesame oil, soy sauce, and grated ginger.

2. Serve over a bed of brown rice or cauliflower rice with steamed broccoli.

10. Mushroom and Spinach Stuffed Chicken Breast:

- Ingredients:

- Chicken breasts

- Mushrooms, chopped

- Fresh spinach

- Garlic, minced

- Goat cheese (optional)

- Preparation:

1. Sauté mushrooms and garlic until softened. Add spinach and cook until wilted.

2. Cut a pocket into each chicken breast and stuff with the mushroom-spinach mixture.

3. Bake until chicken is cooked through.

These dinner recipes provide a variety of flavorful and thyroid-friendly options. Adjust ingredients and portions based on individual preferences and dietary needs, and consult with healthcare professionals for personalized advice.

CHAPTER 6: SNACK AND DESSERT RECIPES

These five nutrient-dense, Hashimoto-friendly snack and dessert recipes will help you maintain the health of your thyroid. Don't forget to modify these recipes according to dietary requirements and personal preferences:

1. Energy-Boosting Nut Mix:

Ingredients:

- 1/2 cup almonds
- 1/2 cup walnuts
- 1/4 cup pumpkin seeds
- 1/4 cup dried goji berries
- 1/4 teaspoon cinnamon

Preparation:

1. In a bowl, combine the goji berries, pumpkin seeds, walnuts, and almonds.

2. Add a sprinkle of cinnamon and mix thoroughly.

2. Greek Yogurt and Berry Parfait:

Ingredients:

- 1 cup Greek yogurt (or dairy-free alternative)
- 1/2 cup mixed berries (e.g., blueberries, strawberries)
- 1 tablespoon chia seeds
- 1 tablespoon honey or maple syrup

Preparation:

1. Arrange mixed berries, Greek yogurt, and chia seeds in a glass or bowl.

2. Drizzle with maple syrup or honey.

3. *Avocado Chocolate Mousse:*

Ingredients:

- 2 ripe avocados
- 1/4 cup cocoa powder
- 1/4 cup maple syrup
- 1 teaspoon vanilla extract

Preparation:

1. Fill a glass or bowl with mixed berries, Greek yogurt, and chia seeds.

2. Drizzle with honey or maple syrup.

4. Baked Apple Slices with Cinnamon:

Ingredients:

- 2 apples, thinly sliced
- 1 tablespoon coconut oil
- 1 teaspoon cinnamon
- 1 tablespoon almond butter (optional)

Preparation:

1. Combine cinnamon and melted coconut oil with apple slices.

2. Bake the apples for tenderness.

3. If preferred, drizzle with almond butter.

5. Coconut Chia Seed Pudding:

Ingredients:

- 2 tablespoons chia seeds
- 1/2 cup coconut milk
- 1/4 teaspoon vanilla extract
- 1/4 cup shredded coconut
- Fresh berries for topping

Preparation:

1. In a container, combine the chia seeds, coconut milk, and vanilla extract.

2. Keep chilled for many hours or overnight.

3. Before serving, sprinkle fresh berries and shredded coconut over top.

These recipes for snacks and desserts provide a harmony of tastes and nutrition to promote thyroid function. Depending on dietary requirements and personal preferences, modify the ingredients and serving sizes. Seek individual counsel from healthcare professionals at all times.

Conclusion

Finally, this cookbook of Hashimoto diet recipes offers a wide variety of satisfying and tasty dishes designed to promote thyroid health. In order to support the management of Hashimoto's disease and enhance general wellbeing, each dish places an emphasis on nutrient-dense ingredients and intelligent combinations.

Adopting this nutritional strategy gives people with Hashimoto's disease access to a variety of meals that are intended to lower inflammation, balance hormones, and improve thyroid function. These recipes, which range from nutrient-dense breakfasts to filling meals and healthy snacks, are delicious and versatile, and they also meet the special requirements of people with Hashimoto's disease.

This cookbook functions as a guide in addition to providing recipes, stressing nutrient-rich options, raising awareness of trigger foods, and encouraging mindful eating practices. It's important to comprehend how food affects health and symptom management in addition to the nutrients.

Although adopting and adjusting to this diet has its obstacles, the benefits are life-changing. People who take control of their eating can feel more energized, have fewer symptoms, and have a fresh lease on life. Keep in mind that progress—small, steady steps toward improved health—rather than perfection—is the aim.

Remember that this cookbook is a tool, a travel partner on your path to better health, as you set out on your culinary voyage. Accept the variety of tastes, play around with the components, and customize this diet to suit your needs. Every action you take to put your health first is a significant act of empowerment and self-care. Your dedication to provide your body with the right foods with these Hashimoto diet recipes opens the door to a future filled with health and vibrancy.

CONTACT US

Dear Reader,

If you have any questions, need further clarification, or require assistance with any aspect of the book, please do not hesitate to reach out to me. I am more than happy to provide additional insights, address your queries, or simply engage in a meaningful discussion.

Feel free to contact me at: IsabelleHartleyBooks@gmail.com. Your feedback and inquiries are always welcome.

FREE 30 DAYS MEAL PLANNER

FREE 30Days Meal Planner, a priceless extra to get you started on the path to a more organized and healthy living. This meticulously curated planner is made to make meal planning easier, save you time, and help you meet your nutritional objectives. Having a month's worth of recipes makes it simpler than ever to stick to your diet goals. Prepare to enjoy the advantages of this wonderful resource! Scan the QR Code below now.